My Sepsis Journey

By

Kim Smith

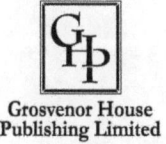

Grosvenor House
Publishing Limited

All rights reserved
Copyright © Kim Smith, 2019

The right of Kim Smith to be identified as the author of this
work has been asserted in accordance with Section 78
of the Copyright, Designs and Patents Act 1988

The book cover is copyright to Kim Smith

This book is published by
Grosvenor House Publishing Ltd
Link House
140 The Broadway, Tolworth, Surrey, KT6 7HT.
www.grosvenorhousepublishing.co.uk

This book is sold subject to the conditions that it shall not, by way of
trade or otherwise, be lent, resold, hired out or otherwise circulated
without the author's or publisher's prior consent in any form of binding or
cover other than that in which it is published and
without a similar condition including this condition being imposed
on the subsequent purchaser.

This book is a work of fiction. Any resemblance to
people or events, past or present, is purely coincidental.

A CIP record for this book
is available from the British Library

ISBN 978-1-78623-585-5

Chapter 1

I had two businesses I was a mobile hairdresser and also ran an events decorating business. I loved doing both, I started as a Saturday girl at the age of thirteen at a salon five minutes from home, I worked the first Saturday and when the next one came round I didn't want to go. I remember asking my mum to ring them and tell them but she insisted I should go in and if I still didn't like it to tell them at the end of the day, I was there for almost three years but went on and qualified as a hairdresser which I was still doing until I lost my limbs, which was forty years in the trade I'd still be working now if I had hands, because my wheelchair wouldn't stop me.

As for the event decorating I loved doing it, mostly weddings and birthday parties doing chair covers and balloons, they absolutely transformed a dull room into a stunning room, I got the same buzz from a messy head of hair when I transformed it into something amazing too, I'd been so busy working it was time to start slowing down a bit and relaxing I couldn't wait to cut down work and get to the sun.

I was in Spain with my husband enjoying the relaxation of not rushing around and having a really nice rest, I used to work seven days a week. We met up with friends in Spain and went for a lovely Indian meal in a neighbouring town, the food was great and so was the company. We were all laughing and joking and enjoying our meals. The next day I started to think I might have a kidney infection when I was getting pain in my left side, just above my waist. The pain was getting really bad by the following day so I decided to go to the local hospital, hoping they would speak more English than the doctors in town and do more tests.

We went to the hospital and with my little bit of Spanish I managed to tell them I had back pain, pointing to the area saying here, presuming they would investigate. I really don't understand why they didn't do more investigation they just X-rayed my back and said nothing was broken, I was just sent away.

It was the twenty-seventh of November 2017 so the fact I was shivering with a blanket around me was understandable it was winter after all, I had extremely cold hands and feet, so Steve, my husband, made a hot water bottle to put under my feet, I had two pairs of socks on and thick sheepskin slippers, I became very breathless but I have asthma so thought it was due to the weather. Then I noticed my speech was slurred when I spoke but didn't think much of it.

The next day I felt really unwell so did a Google Translate on my phone to show the doctor at the local surgery, I translated, "I think I have a urine infection and a temperature." Steve took me to the town medical centre; I remember struggling to walk and having to shuffle my feet. By this time, I was definitely really unwell. I showed the doctor, apparently, I had to give a urine sample, he gave me an injection in my bottom but I don't know what it was and gave us a prescription for antibiotics, we went to the local chemist. Unfortunately, they didn't have any in stock and told us to come back the next day.

We went home but I don't remember much about what I did except I remember that I didn't eat as I was feeling unwell and didn't want anything, I think I went to bed early. I woke at around 4 a.m feeling incredibly unwell and knew I needed to go straight to hospital. I woke Steve, told him and he brought the car round from the side of the villa to the front and up the slope so I didn't have to walk far. At the hospital Steve pulled up at the front and porters came out with a wheelchair, I was taken straight through. This time there was a nurse that spoke English asking me questions about previous operations and medication I took.

I was taken to the intensive care unit (ICU) and put straight into an induced coma. I had a tracheotomy and was placed on life support. A doctor gave my dressing gown, pyjamas and all my jewellery to Steve saying, "She won't be needing these she could die." I can only imagine the absolute fear and confusion he was felt, he had expected that he was taking me to hospital that they would give me some antibiotics and send me home, but to hear that I could die and not to be able to speak the language to ask the staff any questions and without anyone to support him!

Steve went back to the villa and phoned my girls; they phoned my mum and my sister who tried frantically to get flights. There was nothing available from Luton so they had to travel to Gatwick and my two daughters and my mum flew out late that afternoon. They were all frantic my mum had her iPad in her hand luggage, which airport security needed to check, at which point she lost her temper saying, "My daughter is in a coma I need to get my flight," or something to that effect, she must have been going out of her mind, I know I would be if it was one of my daughters.

They arrived at Alicante and our friends Alyson and Kevin were there to meet them. They have strict visiting times in ICU so no one could visit until the next day; they arrived to see me the next morning, they could only see me through what has been described as a fast-food drive-through window. They could only see me and talk to me through this window, which was awful for them. They just wanted to be with me hold my hand cuddle me but they couldn't, it was unbearable for them. They were not allowed into the room until lunchtime. When Becki came in to see me, she pulled back the sheet to hold my hand and she knew right at that moment that I would lose my hands because they were purple, my mum was distraught.

They were only allowed to visit three times a day, morning through a window, afternoon and evening in the room and for just half an hour. The day after my girls and mum arrived my daughter-in-law and sister arrived, Kevin picked them up from the airport, at least with all these women he was getting fed, he'd never cooked meals – I did all the cooking.

One day, about a week in, my kidneys had started to fail and I was put onto kidney dialysis and a tracheotomy was fitted. After two weeks in ICU I had had dialysis for about two weeks when one day one of the nurses turned to my daughter and said, "She pee on own." My daughter repeated this to be sure and the nurse said, "Yes." My daughter was so happy and excited she knew this was a good sign.

When sepsis goes into septic shock that's when vital organs like kidneys start to shut down, it often means you are close to death. I was still in the coma but they visited everyday they played my wedding songs to me, and those of mine and my sisters favourite song dance we'd listened to with my father. We lost our dad when he was just fifty-four, I've never felt such pain, he had a heart attack and died in his sleep.

In the Alicante hospital they would sit and talk to me telling jokes, anything hoping it would help me wake up. One day I did open my eyes a little, my sister had said something and I raised an eyebrow as if to let them know I was listening – not that I remember anything of this.

While in Spain the family visited every day taking it in turns to be with me but it was so hard for them all but especially for my mum, I think it aged her, worrying that her daughter was going to die!

Chapter 2

A few days of after arriving in Spain my girls and Steve sat talking and crying saying they felt they needed to prepare for the worst, I'd been given just six hours to live and things weren't looking good, there was no improvement and they were all worried sick. But time went on and week after week I was still fighting to live, I clearly wasn't going to give up easily. I was in ICU in Spain for six weeks, when my youngest daughter went through my phone and found my travel insurance, she'd had a conversation with them telling them the situation to which they had replied, "We can't foresee why she can't travel back on a commercial airline."

My daughter lost it with them saying, "How on earth is she supposed to get on a plane with all her life-support equipment and everything?" She told them that they were stupid! Well, with that they checked and came back to say they were sending an air ambulance to take me back to the UK.

It was the sixth of January 2018, a doctor from Germany arrived to bring me home, he said to my husband, "I don't know how they work here, but we don't work like this if I don't take her today, she will be dead within two days." He explained to Steve that there was a risk with going up in the air and coming back down due to the air pressure but he would take my life into his hands.

He was in the room for ages taking all their machines off me and attaching his machines up ready to transport me to Alicante Airport for the flight back to Luton and then on to Milton Keynes Hospital who were waiting to receive me in the department of critical care (DOCC).

My girls were there waiting for me to arrive they said I was in what looked like a body bag, the staff took me into a side room and got me all wired up, then took my girls into an office and said, "We want to warn you the next forty-eight hours are critical she's in a really bad way."

I had a bad pressure sore on my bottom and one which was a grade 4 on the back of my head which they showed my girls so that they knew they'd been caused in Spain, I'm very lucky to only have a small scar there now where hair will never grow again.

After three weeks in the DOCC they started waking me up, I don't remember much of it because of delirium due to the drugs and the coma. I had really bad delirium, I thought my husband was having an affair with a man and I told my girls he was gay, anyone who knows my husband knows this is definitely not true! I thought he was having an affair with one of the nurses too, I also thought there was a cat at the end of my bed – I'm petrified of cats and started screaming for them to remove it. My family had put pictures up on the wall and I thought they were people coming to attack me. I also said, "Let's go and have a barbeque on the beach in Australia." And that I needed to go and get a takeaway as the hospital food was disgusting. I was moved down to Ward 2 after a week and I thought they were having a party on the ward, and that I'd seen them bringing in alcohol and they had a karaoke. Strange how the brain makes you believe it's all true even though none of it was true!

While I was in the DOCC my girls warned me that the doctor was coming to see me about my hands and legs, I knew they were black so I knew they were dead and I couldn't lift them it was as though they were fixed to the bed. The doctor came in and I was told that if I didn't agree to having the amputations, they suspected the gangrene would take over my body. He said, "I need to talk to you about your limbs, I'm afraid we are going to have to amputate."

I replied, "That's fine, I can see you need to do it, so just do it as soon as possible please!" I don't think the doctor was expecting my response but I felt the sooner it was done the sooner I could get home. For my amputations I was transferred to Bedford and a couple of days later, on the ninth of February 2018, I was taken to theatre. They had asked my daughter to sign the consent form and had said they intended to amputate one leg and debride my arms. My daughter got a call after a while, at first she panicked, thinking something was wrong but they said that everything was going better than expected and there had been minimal blood loss so they asked her if she would consent to both legs being amputated, she agreed to this. So, when I was taken to intensive care, I had had all four limbs removed the operation had gone so well that they had managed to remove them all in one go. My girls met the doctor going into the ICU and he assured them they'd managed to amputate all four limbs in one go. When I woke, I was happy they'd managed to do it in one go I didn't really want to have four separate operations.

After two weeks I had to have further surgery to close my hand stumps, they'd left them open in case

I decided I'd like a hand transplant. They asked me and I thought about it but just didn't feel I could handle looking at someone else's hands, not only that but I'd have had to take medication and lots of it to stop them from being rejected and there was no guarantee that they wouldn't be rejected at some point so I decided it wasn't for me.

After the operations my leg stumps had staples for about three weeks until they were removed, they healed really quickly. But my arms took a long time it was at least three months, because they'd been debrided and they were like really severe burns with no skin on. They had to be redressed every day but gradually I could see them improving while I laid in bed for three months in Bedford Hospital in a side room. My family would come every day to help look after me and feed me as I couldn't do anything for myself, pretty much all the staff where lovely except for two really horrible bank staff who really upset me. When I rang the bell a couple of times, they told me how busy they were and that they couldn't keep dropping everything to come to me. If I could have done anything for myself I would have done. I only asked if I couldn't wait or needed help urgently, it really upset me. The nursing sister told me that that was what they were paid for saying, "I don't care if you ring the bell 500 times a day, if you need something you ring them and if they don't do it tell me." She was so lovely, thankfully my family did pretty much everything so I rarely rang for anything.

The night I was taken to Bedford Hospital my Becki came with me, she slept on the floor next to me. At one point she felt a spider on her so jumped up and tried to sleep in the upright chair, she was absolutely amazing.

Her employer was amazing too, she took almost six months off to be with me every day. Gemma would come too they would bring my mum and my sister; I always had a member of family with me during the day. I remember Steve coming in one day and, apparently, I thought he hadn't visited and said, "Oh you've turned up then!"

On the twenty-seventh of March I was taken to Queen Mary's Hospital in Roehampton for an assessment, I met physiotherapists, occupational therapists (OTs), doctors and nurses of the large team that would look after me once I arrived to stay there, the assessment went well and I returned to Bedford to wait for a bed at Roehampton. At Bedford, in the meantime, I was supposed to be have physiotherapy but they rarely had time, I was lucky if I got half an hour a week. On those occasions they got me a wheelchair and I was just hoisted into it once a week and left. What a difference at Roehampton, straightaway I was in the gym twice a day five days a week and was learning how to move again. My first session in the gym was on the eighth of May 2018, I was hoisted at this point onto a plinth, I began by doing stretches then used an exercise ball for balance. I had to learn how to shuffle, it's strange how you don't know how to do it and have to learn it all over again but by the end of my first day I was off like a rocket and they were really happy with me, they said that I did much better than they had expected I would on my first day!

Chapter 3

On the fifteenth of May I'd been up all night with tummy pain, I thought I had a urine infection but it turned out my catheter was blocked so after it was flushed, I spent the day in bed sleeping. I was so upset that I had missed the gym session but the next day I was up and, in the gym, doing all my exercises and shuffling up and down the plinth, I used small stools for support at first but gradually I didn't need them. I managed to go backwards into my wheelchair from the plinth on the sixteenth without the small stools and as I was getting on so well that I knew it wouldn't be long before I would be able to go home with my family again. On the twenty-seventh of May I had a visit from my daughter and my mum and I showed them how I could shuffle on my bed at that stage. I was so proud but so were they watching me do this they were smiling from ear to ear.

On the thirtieth of May the OT said she was amazed at how well I was doing and it was all due to my great core strength. My goal was to get home, that's why I was working so hard, I didn't tell her that but I'm sure she knew!

I started doing training on the computer to use a NHS myoelectric hand, my test score was the highest of anyone the OT had worked with before. I said that I thought it was possibly because I was a hairdresser and was used to using these muscles in my arm when cutting hair. I absolutely loved doing these practice sessions it was fun making the muscles in my arm move to make the car on the screen move between gaps.

On the fourth of June I was practicing transferring using a banana board I had to go across a wide gap between the plinth and my wheelchair to practice getting in and out of the car, it was scary at first but I soon managed it without a problem. I was allowed a weekend home visit that weekend and I was so excited. A special bed was being delivered for me and I was so excited to be seeing my dogs after seven long months and they were very excited to see me to. It was a very busy time as lots of friends and family came to see me and my GP made a home visit too, she was so lovely.

My daughter and Mum came to visit me and Gemma put me in the wheelchair so she could do my hair colour for me. I was desperate for this to be done as nearly all my colour had grown out, I hadn't seen my natural colour since I was thirteen. I don't like my hair dark so, bless her, she did my hi-lights, washed it off and dried it. It was a lovely sunny day so we went to sit in the garden, it was lovely to get outside. I remember the first time outside after my operation was with my youngest daughter at Bedford Hospital, they'd hoisted me into a wheelchair and Becki took me into the garden, I'd been stuck in bed for months and it was so good to get into that wheelchair and go and sit in the sun. At that time, I couldn't sit for long but even the fifteen minutes or so that I managed was a huge boost, so much better than being stuck in a hospital room all the time.

My best friend visited me several times while I was in Bedford, we always did each other's hair but mine was so messy now. I had a huge gap at the back of my head, I'd been brought back from Spain with the grade 4 pressure sore on the back of my head but my hair had got so long on top and I had long straggling bits at the back, so I'd asked her to bring her scissors and cut it for me. Afterwards it made me feel better just knowing my hair looked better, she's been such a good friend over the years we've known each other since I was about fifteen years old, we used to go everywhere together. I was a bridesmaid when she got married, I introduced her to her husband I'd been friends with him and his family for years, we were both there for each other when our marriages broke down, our children are fairly close in ages but she had her first about two years before me. My eldest and her youngest are six months apart, they have been best friends since birth it's lovely to have such a good friend as Chris, and for months she wouldn't let me pay her for cutting my hair, even though she was so busy that I would have had trouble getting an appointment.

On the sixth of June 2018 I found the bionic arm I'd seen on Davina McCall's show, "This time next year." On the show there was a girl called Tilly who'd lost her hands due to meningitis, the prosthetic hands were amazing. After much searching, I became the first quadruple amputee to be fitted with one of Open Bionic's Hero Arms, it's truly amazing and I love it. My story has been in the *Sunday People* a few times. Once was after I received my Hero Arm they were happy to hear my fundraising had helped reach enough to buy my first arm.

I was so very lucky that my daughter set up my first GoFundMe page to raise the money for my Hero Arm. A lady had contacted my girls, she knew lots of my old school friends she arranged a disco while I was still in Bedford Hospital her name was Lorraine, she raised about £1,700, I think. What a lovely person to do such a wonderful thing. Then my mum said her friend had been talking to someone that knew me and he wanted to do a disco for me. I'd known Martin and his brothers and mum for many years as I used to do his mum's hair and I had worked for his sister-in-law for a few years too. I think he raised just under £1,000 so the fundraising went pretty quickly. The *Sunday People* made a video of me in Bedford Hospital and took photos for the paper, telling readers about my story. I was so lucky people were helping raise money for me, I was so grateful and the paper has done a couple of stories now, following up with when I got my arm and when I went and did my indoor skydive, that was fantastic!

On the thirteenth of June I was discharged from Roehampton Hospital where I'd been expecting to stay for twelve weeks but I did so well I was discharged early. It was so good to be home with my family at long last and to be my dogs and not to have to go back to hospital again! Although it was good to get out, I hate being starred at, I don't mind children but adults stare and they don't see me looking at them because they are too busy starring at my missing limbs, I sometimes get very upset by it, I've been known to shout out, "Has no one ever told you it's rude to stare?"

On the twenty-second of June 2018 I won the Milton Keynes Inspirational Woman Award, everyone was always telling me I was inspirational but I felt like I was just me, I'd just come out of hospital I wasn't used to sitting in my wheelchair for long and I was more comfortable on my bed, so I didn't go to the award presentation. A friend called Corina was going the presentation, as she'd been nominated for the Most Charitable Business. She does so much for charity I'm not surprised that she won that award. She offered to collect mine if I won, and told me to write down what I'd like to say if I won. I was blown away because I won the Inspirational Woman Award and her daughter Casey read out my speech. Corina had loaned me costumes from her business so friends could dress up and raise money for me, she's a very special lady who does so much to help others. Many people have said that they couldn't have coped with what I went through but I'm sure we all can if we have to. It has definitely life changing and very challenging at times but I'm up for the challenge as long as my amazing family and husband are supporting me, without them I couldn't have done this they are my strength and they encourage me to do things.

On the twenty-seventh of June I went to Burton upon Trent, to a company called Dorset Orthopaedics, who took a cast of my stumps for my Hero Arm, which Open Bionics supply. It was amazing I tried how the arm worked and my daughter videoed me picking up a can of coke and pretending to drink from it. I was so excited about getting hands again I've always been so crafty the thought of never being able to do things would have driven me crazy. I've been very happy to get just one for now. I also have an NHS one, it's very heavy and it's not as good. Even the OT was impressed with the tests I did to compare both arms. The Hero Arm won by a mile, so much more movement and lighter to, my grandson loves it he says I'm his robot nanny. Bless him, he's only five and will probably never remember me with hands and legs which is sad, but I'm happy to be alive!

My Hero Arm was £15,000 with a five-year accidental warranty I had to take the warranty out after spending so much on the arm just in case I have an accident to me it's worth every penny!

On the fourth of July I ordered my wheelchair and upgraded it. As I will be in a wheelchair for the rest of my life I chose a Rise & Tilt. I can rise to go up high for when I'm able to start cooking again and tilt when I need to take the pressure off my bottom a little or on long journeys in the Mobility vehicle, I also chose a padded back rest and head rest. It cost an extortionate amount almost £2,500 just for a few upgrades but it's worth it to have a wonderful comfortable chair to get around in. I was promised it in eight days but it took months I had so many excuses I certainly wouldn't recommend the company I bought it from.

I was contacted by a friend, who said that she had had some building work done and she told the builders about me. They said that they wanted to do something to help, two lovely guys. They decided to do a sponsored bike ride from Milton Keynes to Oxford. On the day of the ride it was pouring with rain so they stopped at a family member's in Oxford. After having something to eat and drink and drying off they set off again but half way back it was raining so heavily that they had to admit defeat and give up. With such bad weather I didn't blame them but they tried so hard, I was very grateful to them to do that for a complete stranger, it was so kind.

On the first of August I got my Hero Arm. My grandson was so happy – I could do fist bumps with him – with my robot hand. as he called it. I was over the moon and it didn't take me long to start using it, brushing my hair and teeth, eating, putting on make-up it's fabulous!

On the sixth of August I got an infection on my left stump and went to A&E, they were brilliant, as soon as I said, "I'm worried I've got an infection and lost my limbs due to sepsis." Within ten minutes they called me into the triage room and had me on intravenous antibiotics I was then taken to a small ward off A&E to wait to see a doctor. After several hours they'd changed shifts and forgotten to tell anyone about me. My daughter told them and they dealt with me and let me go home, I was told I'd have to go back to Bedford to see my surgeon as he thought the bone was infected because it was out of the skin, so I was referred urgently and was operated on within the week. Luckily it wasn't too bad and within two weeks it was all healed although I panicked when they first told me because it was possible that I might have lost a lot more of my arm!

So far on my journey I've got arms and now I've decided to try for stubbies. Stubbies aren't really legs they have a rocker on the bottom of a socket, these can take a long time to get to the stage where you are able to walk. Once you can walk, if you want to, you can gradually build up the length on the legs, I was told, at an inch at a time. This is for double above knee amputees, like me not for a single or a below knee amputee, I've had my legs cast and I'm waiting for my sockets to be ready for the next stage. To build up my muscles to help with the walking I'm going to start swimming to add to the daily physio at home and once a week at Stanmore (where I've been transferred to as it's much closer to home).

A few weeks ago (seventeenth of April 2019) I went to Netheravon Army Air Corps barracks near Salisbury, to do a skydive. Since surviving death, I have decided I'd like to do anything and everything I can as an amputee and I had found this air base offering skydiving. They were absolutely brilliant with me and I had the time of my life I loved every minute of it and I'm now looking for other things to do.

I've found a centre down in Exmoor, they do everything you can think of and certainly things I'd like to try: horse riding, canoeing, abseiling and so much more I'm really looking forward to going for a weekend to try these things.

My passion, since surviving sepsis is to tell everyone about sepsis. I'm a volunteer for the Sepsis Trust UK, and I've given talks for them. I've also given a talk for doctors and nurses at a hotel in Milton Keynes, this was great because they were medical staff and I was able to show them the pictures of my black limbs and, believe me, even doctors gasped because it's not often they see anything as severe as that. I did another talk recently at the hospital for Health Care Assistants (HCAs) and again I got gasps, I'm happy to tell my story to anyone, all I hope is that it might help to save lives. So far I've had a few people say if it hadn't been for me they wouldn't have known about sepsis and a loved one might have died but they took them to hospital, that's such amazing news, eventually everyone, even medical staff, will know the symptoms of sepsis and more people will survive but we still have a lot of work to do.

Chapter 4

Useful information has been provided by the Sepsis Trust UK and they have kindly given permission for it to be reproduced here.

Sepsis can leave you with lots of side effects it's called Post-Sepsis Syndrome (PSS)

PHYSICAL SYMPTOMS OF PSS:

- Lethargy/excessive tiredness
- Poor mobility/muscle weakness
- Breathlessness/chest pains
- Swollen limbs (excessive fluid in the tissues)
- Joint and muscle pains
- Insomnia
- Hair loss
- Dry/flaking skin and nails
- Taste changes
- Poor appetite
- Changes in vision
- Changes in the sensation in limbs
- Repeated infections from the original site or a new site
- Reduced kidney function
- Feeling cold
- Excessive sweating.

PSYCHOLOGICAL AND EMOTIONAL SYMPTOMS OF PSS:

- Anxiety/fear of sepsis recurring
- Depression
- Flashbacks
- Nightmares
- Insomnia (due to stress or anxiety)
- Post-Traumatic Stress Disorder (PTSD)
- Poor concentration
- Short-term memory loss
- Mood swings.

WHAT TREATMENT IS AVAILABLE?

There is no specific treatment for PSS, but most people will get better with time. In the meantime, it's a case of managing the individual problems and looking after yourself while you are recovering.

Tell your family and friends about PSS, explain how you feel and give them information to read so they can understand what you're going through. It will help you all get through this difficult time.

Not all doctors know about PSS, so it may be helpful to take a hospital booklet with you or to print out this information. It is important that your doctor assesses your symptoms and excludes any other causes of the problems. Your doctor may refer you to a different professional to help manage individual PSS problems, such as a pain specialist to manage your pain, a counsellor or psychiatrist to manage mental health and emotional problems, or a physio or an OT to manage fatigue.

If you are struggling with your recovery, you can call a helpline and speak to a member of a support team. These are trained nurses with an understanding of sepsis and the problems that can occur during recovery.

Above all, remind yourself that, horrible as PSS is, you're not alone, and these problems are part of the recovery process. Sometimes you have to look back to where you started to see how far you have come.

I suffer from anxiety about sepsis reoccurring, I'm on antidepressants for depression, I have occasional nightmares, I often don't sleep well, I definitely have very poor concentration and I have severe memory problems but it's getting better. The mood swings are reducing but if I flip, I really flip and I'm a nightmare, I don't like it but it is what it is, hopefully it will all get better in time, I suffer some of the physical symptoms too, but thankfully nothing to often.

Chapter 5

Sepsis is a serious complication of an infection. Without quick treatment, sepsis can lead to multiple-organ failure and death.

Sepsis symptoms in babies and children

Go straight to A&E or call 999 if your child has any of these symptoms:

- looks mottled, bluish or pale
- is very lethargic or difficult to wake
- feels abnormally cold to touch
- is breathing very fast
- has a rash that does not fade when you press it
- has a fit or convulsion.

Get medical advice urgently from NHS 111

If your child has any of the symptoms listed below, is getting worse or is sicker than you'd expect (even if their temperature falls), trust your instincts and seek medical advice urgently on NHS 111.

Temperature

- a temperature over 38C in babies under three months

- a temperature over 39C in babies aged three to six months
- any high temperature in a child who cannot be encouraged to show interest in anything
- a low temperature (below 36C – check three times in a ten-minute period).

Breathing

- finding it much harder to breathe than normal – looks like hard work
- making "grunting" noises with every breath
- cannot say more than a few words at once (for older children who normally talk)
- breathing that obviously "pauses".

Toilet/nappies

- not had a wee or wet nappy for twelve hours

Eating and drinking

- new baby under one month old with no interest in feeding
- not drinking for more than eight hours (when awake)
- bile-stained (green), bloody or black vomit/sick.

Activity and body

- soft spot on a baby's head is bulging
- eyes look "sunken"
- child cannot be encouraged to show interest in anything
- baby is floppy

- weak, "whining" or continuous crying in a younger child
- older child who's confused
- not responding or very irritable
- stiff neck, especially when trying to look up and down.

Sepsis symptoms in older children and adults

Early symptoms

Early symptoms of sepsis may include:

- a high temperature or a low body temperature
- chills and shivering
- a fast heartbeat
- problems or changes to your breathing
- feeling or acting differently from normal – you do not seem your usual self.

Many of the symptoms of sepsis are also associated with meningitis.

The first symptoms are often fever, vomiting, a headache and feeling unwell.

Septic shock

In some cases, symptoms of more severe sepsis or when your blood pressure drops to a dangerously low level, develop soon after.

These can include:

- feeling dizzy or faint
- a change in mental state, such as confusion or disorientation

- diarrhoea
- nausea and vomiting
- slurred speech
- severe muscle pain
- severe breathlessness
- less urine production than normal – for example, not urinating for a day
- cold, clammy and pale or mottled skin
- loss of consciousness.

When to get medical help

Seek medical advice urgently from NHS 111 if you have recently had an infection or injury and have possible early signs of sepsis.

If sepsis is suspected, you'll usually be referred to hospital for further diagnosis and treatment.

Severe sepsis and septic shock are medical emergencies. If you think you or someone in your care has one of these conditions, go straight to A&E or call 999.

Tests to diagnose sepsis

Sepsis is often diagnosed based on simple measurements such as your temperature, heart rate and breathing rate. You may need to have a blood test.

Other tests can help determine the type of infection, where it's located and which body functions have been affected.

These include:

- urine or stool samples
- a small sample of tissue, skin or fluid being taken from the affected area for testing (a wound culture)

- taking a sample of saliva, phlegm or mucus (respiratory secretion testing)
- blood pressure tests
- imaging studies, such as an X-Ray, ultrasound scan or computerised tomography (CT) Scan.

Treatments for sepsis

If sepsis is detected early and has not affected vital organs yet, it may be possible to treat the infection at home with antibiotics.

Most people who have sepsis detected at this stage make a full recovery.

Almost all people with severe sepsis and septic shock require admission to hospital. Some people may require admission to an ICU.

Because of problems with vital organs, people with severe sepsis are likely to be very ill and the condition can be fatal.

But sepsis is treatable if it's identified and treated quickly, and in most cases leads to a full recovery with no lasting problems.

Recovering from sepsis

Some people make a full recovery fairly quickly.

The amount of time it takes to fully recover from sepsis varies, depending on:

- the severity of the sepsis
- the person's overall health
- how much time was spent in hospital?
- whether treatment was needed in an ICU.

Some people experience long-term physical or psychological problems during their recovery period, such as:

- feeling lethargic or excessively tired
- muscle weakness
- swollen limbs or joint pain
- chest pain or breathlessness.

These long-term problems are known as PPS. Not everyone experiences these problems.

Who's at risk

There are around 250,000 cases of sepsis a year in the UK according to the UK Sepsis Trust. At least 46,000 people die every year as a result of the condition.

Anyone can develop sepsis after an injury or minor infection, although some people are more at risk of sepsis.

This includes:

- babies and elderly people
- people who are frail or have a weakened immune system
- people who have recently had surgery.

Sepsis, septicaemia and blood poisoning

Although sepsis is often referred to as either blood poisoning or septicaemia, these terms refer to the invasion of bacteria into the bloodstream.

Sepsis can affect multiple organs or the entire body, even without blood poisoning or septicaemia.

Sepsis can also be caused by viral or fungal infections, although bacterial infections are by far the most common cause.

Chapter 6

On Thursday the seventeenth of June 2019 I went to Stanmore for my physiotherapy appointment but also had an appointment with my prosthetist. I was excited because I'd had my casts done a couple of weeks before so I knew this meant I'd be trying them on, we arrived early and it wasn't long before I was called in. He put my liners on then the casts, I then had to stand up so he could check them, he took them off made some adjustments and then got me to stand again, I can't tell you how good it felt to stand after eighteen months of sitting, I can't wait to start practicing walking it's all so real now. The doctor who did my amputations said I'd never walk again and I wasn't too worried at first, I was alive and that's what meant more to me, but I started gaining a lot of weight just sitting so I knew that if I could walk it would help. Then I heard about stubbies, you start with short ones of these and gradually build up their length, at the moment I'm concentrating on using stubbies and I'm not worried about normal length legs yet, but I don't say never as I might want to have a longer leg in the future, one step at a time, literally lol!

After my fitting with my sockets my daughter and I had some lunch before my physio. Appointment. That day it was in the swimming pool as I'd mentioned I'd like to try swimming again, it was amazing I absolutely loved it, I really was quite anxious beforehand possibly partly because of the weight I'd put on and I was conscious of that and partly because I wasn't sure if I could float or swim without legs. There are special swimming pool wheelchairs, so I transferred onto one of these and they wheeled me down the ramp, at the bottom I edged myself off the chair to hold onto the side. I did exercises bringing my core to pull and push me from the side then held onto the side, scissor kicking my legs, before they got me swimming on my back for a few widths and then lengths. Then they took me to the side again to do some more pulling in and away from the side and scissor kicks and that hour went quickly, so I thought I would let go and swim to the wheelchair. I started all right but then took a nose dive, I managed to flip onto my back thinking I could float again when thankfully they grabbed me, I won't try that again. I need more time but I loved it and can't wait to try going in a pool again.

A while ago I became a volunteer for the Sepsis Trust, since having sepsis and not knowing the symptoms I've made it my mission to warn everyone since I started writing on my Facebook page, which is called Kim's Chance, I regularly post about sepsis. I've joined lots of different groups and I was asked by my GP surgery if I'd talk to doctors and nurses at a conference in a hotel in Milton Keynes of course I jumped at the chance, my daughter helped me do a PowerPoint presentation and I sent it to a lady at the surgery which was helping, for her approval, she loved it. I now use this for all my presentations it's a very powerful presentation with the graphic pictures of my very black limbs, I get gasps even from medical staff. I'm hoping that it makes them remember my story and it helps to save lives, I had someone not so long ago message my Kim's Chance page saying if it hadn't been for my posts on my page her boyfriend would be dead but she'd remembered what I'd posted and rang the 111 service, they sent an ambulance and got him to hospital in time, she thanked me and praised me, so I'm happy I've maybe helped towards saving someone's life. Now I've stepped up my mission with help from Melissa at the Sepsis Trust, I have contacted the Lead Sepsis Nurse who I did a talk for again recently and asked her if she knew of anywhere I could help further. She's arranging for me to meet with midwives next, I posted on Facebook asking if anyone knew of any groups that would like to have me in to give a talk and I've now got two confirmed bookings. I've contacted every school in Milton Keynes by email, a couple have responded but nothing is booked yet, I hope they do. I'm also going into a retirement village

I'm so passionate about trying to warn everyone about sepsis so this doesn't happen to them or worse they die. Most people have heard of sepsis but so many still don't know the symptoms, I was probably the same, I probably thought that it wouldn't happen to me. What I didn't know then was that infection can occur in different places, from a paper cut to a urinary tract infection (UTI) any infected area can lead to an extreme reaction by our immune system which goes into overdrive and causes sepsis

I'm now trying to get as much awareness as possible in the Milton Keynes area and beyond. I won't sit back and do nothing I don't want more families suffering like mine have. My family here all been amazing helping me,

I've always been so independent I hated asking for help but I don't have a choice now as I need help. My husband had never done any cooking I always did that, I even preferred to cook than to go out for a meal! But my husband has to cook now he doesn't like it and doesn't understand why people like cooking but he's doing amazingly well. I tell him what to do what spices to add, how long to cook things for, kind of like a talking cookery book and he's cooking wonderful meals. I don't know how he's coped with me being like this it's not easy for him and at first I kept telling him to go, I thought he'd be better without the burden I'd become but he's such a wonderful husband he takes such good care of me I'm so very lucky!

I'm very lucky though I've become friends with some lovely people who have lost loved ones to sepsis. One, who was pregnant when her husband became very ill and passed away from sepsis extremely suddenly and another who has lost her son, it breaks my heart seeing how much they are suffering because of sepsis and it pushes me to do more. I'm lucky I'm alive and my story, I guess like the nurse said at Milton Keynes General Hospital, is a powerful story, hopefully people will start remembering the symptoms soon and fewer people will die from it!

Sarah, who is the mummy of Dylan who passed away, also has a page. She uploads daily information about Dylan and sepsis, I didn't know her before but saw her posts, we've become friends and I feel for her and her family. No parent should lose a child it just doesn't bear thinking about the pain that the whole family are suffering. Recently Sarah has had a baby girl and hopefully this will ease her pain and that of her other children just a little bit now. Nothing can replace someone you've lost but I pray it eases their pain, I can only imagine how hard it must be as a mother and grandmother myself. This makes me think about how hard it must have been for my family when I was in the coma especially while I was in Spain and they didn't speak much English to be able to get any questions answered, luckily we knew someone who used to come up and translate so they got updates from time to time but nine weeks of not knowing if I'd live or die, they must have been going out of their minds!

While I was in hospital, I met my first quadruple amputee I think he'd become an amputee about a month before I did and his was also due to sepsis. Then I learned about a boy who lives in Leighton buzzard not far from Milton Keynes, I became friends with his mum and step dad, we've met several times since, the last time was when Kye and I compared our bionic arms. I got mine last August but Kye didn't get his until about February this year (2019) he's such a shy boy – well with adults he is – but not with grandchildren! He had meningitis which turned to sepsis, he's got part of a hand on his right and he's got one below knee and one through knee, I had no idea about what all this meant before but being below knee it's much easier to walk again than it is if you're above knee like I am but where there's a way there's a will there's a way, as they say and I will!

Steph lives near me I kept seeing her posts about sepsis and about how she'd lost her husband to it, on Facebook I started to follow her, we then became friends on Facebook, the poor girl was six months pregnant with their first baby, they were making plans for the baby's arrival and for the rest of their lives as a family. Daniel got poorly and thinking he needed help she got him to hospital (they'd been told by the GP that he had gastroenteritis, I believe) but within no time he deteriorated and passed away, obviously she was bereaved, she'd lost the love of her life her soulmate and she didn't want to carry on without him, but she had to for their beautiful little girl. When Steph had the baby, she was dealt another cruel blow, she had contracted sepsis during her labour and passed it to the baby, they had to spend five days in hospital on antibiotics and poor Jessica had to have a lumber puncture at just one day old!

They were having a three-day Sepsis Awareness session at our local Tesco's where Daniel used to work. We did three days down there fundraising for me as well, so I decided to give her half of what we made, she didn't want to take it but I insisted it was for her and Daniel's beautiful baby daughter for later in life. We meet from time to time and we message each other occasionally, we think of her all the time sepsis is cruel it doesn't care who it hurts, it doesn't care if you know the symptoms or not, it doesn't care if it takes your soulmate, your child, your parent, aunt or uncle we need more awareness to stop it!

On Saturday the eighteenth of May 2019, I went to walk my dog with my husband it was a lovely hot sunny day and although I shouldn't go in the sun for too long, because of my sepsis scars, it was pleasant to get outside in the fresh air and sunshine so we walking down the road. Two little girls were playing, one had a bike the other a scooter, when the youngest one said, "Why don't you have hands?"

I said "I was very poorly from an infection and the doctor had to cut them off so I could live. I haven't got legs either."

She helped me lift my skirt to show her, her dad kept saying sorry and I told him that it was fine I really didn't mind. She was adorable, she said, "It's kinda weird not having hands."

Again, her dad said, "Sorry."

I replied, "But she's right it is weird, I'd never seen anyone without hands before this happened to me."

She chatted to me for ages, it was so lovely, then she asked can I touch them and of course I said she could. Bless her, she felt comfortable enough to want to see if they felt the same, I guess but I was more than happy to let her, I think it's good to talk about it especially to children. Adults probably wonder, so often they stare, I'd far rather they ask just like this beautiful little girl did, I'll never forget her, it was lovely! I think we could all learn a thing or two from children

Chapter 7

When I first came out of hospital I had a care company visiting in twice a day, I hated that I had different people all the time some were rough too, there were always two and one day I lost it, because one was rushing to wash the top end and one the bottom end. I couldn't handle it and freaked out it upset me really badly, after a conversation with my social worker I was told she could go to panel under special circumstances and ask for my daughter to be my carer. They only allow it occasionally but she felt I had a good case; she was so lovely helping me she knew how it upset me. I'd also had another carer who I had to report because I felt very uncomfortable with how she was washing me down below, I couldn't do anything for myself so to feel this uncomfortable was alarming. I refused to let her in to the house again, it really was the last straw, so when my case went to panel, they agreed and my eldest daughter, who works for herself, was able to become my carer.

Never in a million years did I think my children would end up doing what they do for me but they truly are amazing. I split with their dad when I was pregnant with my youngest and he's never wanted to have any contact with them, not that that is what he tells people. I've always worked very hard and given them everything I could, we had a holiday abroad every year and had a great life, they tell me I was their mum and their dad until I met Steve. My eldest daughter was about eight when I met him, I'd started working for his sister in a salon, one day he phoned to speak to her and I answered the phone, later he asked her who had answered the phone and she said the new girl Kim, with that he started phoning every day when I was at work. After two months I said, "You keep phoning me at work it's about time you took me for a drink."

He replied, "I'm in Milton Keynes tonight, give me your address and I'll come and have a coffee with you."

He lived in London, but his two children lived in Milton Keynes and he came up every weekend to see them, that was twenty-two years ago. We dated for five years before moving in together and arranged to get married two years later, we went to Cypress to get married. We married in Paphos Town Hall in 2014 and our friends and family joined us, my two daughters Steve's daughter and my great niece where bridesmaids and Steve's son was best man. Our mums didn't come as they both felt it was too much for them, we had twenty of us altogether the hotel was amazing. I'd found their email and I arranged to have the reception at the hotel, we had canopies and champagne on arrival back at the hotel then we had a break so everyone could relax by the pool followed in the evening with a seven course meal and wine by the pool, it was the most amazing wedding and Steve wanted to do it again.

I've been very lucky he's a kind, generous man and he's been a wonderful dad to my girls and a wonderful husband to me, I really don't tell him this anywhere near often enough.

This September we will have been married for fifteen years and I can honestly say they have been the happiest of my life. I certainly don't know what I'd have done without him these last eighteen months, so far, since becoming a quadruple amputee, I always thought he'd be the one to die first and I didn't think he'd cope if it was me, but thanks to my girls supporting him while I was in the coma and since he's done so remarkably well, I'm extremely proud of him.

The OT at Stanmore said she was going to get me in the kitchen and help me to be able to do more, she would show me different gadgets and ways of doing more in the kitchen using my amazing Hero Arm. With the right tools and gadgets I'm sure I can take over in the kitchen again, but I will probably need help with things as I don't think I'd be able to put things in to the oven, or get them out for that matter!

I'm also very proud of both my daughters they were with me every single day in Milton Keynes and Bedford Hospital until Becki had to go back to work after the three months she had taken off to be with me. They used to feed me to help the nurses and I remember when I first came out of the coma finding the food was really bland, so Becki used to make me spicy curries and chilli con carne, for some reason I just wanted really spicy food, much spicier than I normally ate. I've always liked spicy food, but that is all I wanted. My favourite food is an Indian, I remember in Roehampton telling a Jamaican nurse that I liked spicy food she asked me if I like jerk chicken, I told her that I'd never tried it but I was sure that I would like it. A few days later she brought me lots in, I'd not eaten that evening because the food had been horrible so I ate the lot it was amazing I definitely love jerk chicken now!

Steve knew I was getting very upset not being able to do things for myself and we were living at my daughter's, he was upstairs I was in the front room, I couldn't sleep, I'd be watching TV on my iPad until 1 or 2 a.m. then often I was awake again at 4 a.m. I got a little depressed too, so bless him, he thought it would be good to take me away for a few days. He's never wanted to take a cruise, I think it's because he's not a strong swimmer not that he'd admit that, but he knew I'd always wanted to take one, and knowing it would be hard for me to get on a plane he booked a four-night cruise going to Bruges and Amsterdam. It was wonderful, getting waited on, the food was fabulous we met some lovely people too, we used to go for dinner then go and watch a show, we aren't big drinkers but we'd have a drink with our meal. Every show we watched was great, he had got a really good deal because it was last minute and we had a lovely balcony, not that we could go on it in November as it was too windy and cold. The cabin was comfortable and big enough for me to get around (as I'd heard that cabins could be tiny) obviously purpose-built cabins for disabled people are bigger so there was no problem at all. Now I'm hoping he'll take me again as I'd like to go to Spain and Portugal on a cruise, perhaps he might take me for my sixtieth – I'm working on him!

As I mentioned earlier, I used to be a hairdresser and my hair was my crowning glory, so losing my hands and not being able to do my hair like I used to is a massive thing for me, some days I look in the mirror and have a melt down because my hair is just awful, but my natural curls have come back so I comb it into place and my daughter straightens the top for me. Now I keep it shorter I don't mind that so much, I'm getting pretty good at putting my make-up on with my stumps now and one of these days I'm going to do a live on Facebook to show everyone how I do it. It's getting easier with practice and I used to have make-up on every day, I wouldn't ever let anyone see me without my make-up but I don't seem to mind now. I think surviving death has changed me a lot, I don't have the same fear of things like I did before, I wouldn't have dreamt of doing a skydive but I absolutely loved every second of it, I was not scared or nervous I was just excited.

It's the same when I go to give talks about sepsis, I'm not nervous because I want to warn people just how serious it is and how it needs urgent medical treatment. How if someone is feeling unwell from any infection if they don't get the right treatment urgently, they often die. If people see me and hear how I lost my limbs, I hope it makes them remember me and my story and if they've forgotten the symptoms, they Google them and get treatment I always say, "Just ask could it be sepsis?" Because still not all medical professionals know the symptoms and they are still being trained, this is why my story is shown in the corridor of Milton Keynes Hospital. There's lots of information and I go and talk to staff, slowly all the volunteers are making progress but we still have a lot to do!

I think being a volunteer keeps me busy and by telling my story is a sort of therapy I like doing it. I'm keen to find other ways to help raise awareness too, if you read my book and tell one person about what happened to me and ask them to tell one more person we will increase the awareness out there and save people from dying, I'm not really religious but I do think I was saved because I've got the ability to help increase awareness and I will!

Chapter 8

A while ago I saw my niece, who was a hairdresser but she doesn't work as a hairdresser now, although she still does haircuts for her family, and I said to her "I've got a practically brand-new pair of jowels (hairdressing scissors) at home would you like them?"

It seemed silly leaving them in my wardrobe never being used, bless her she said, "I've still got the old ones you gave me years ago." I had given them to her when she finished her training and I'd brought a new pair,

I had said, "There's one condition though, I need my hair cut, so would you cut it for me please."

I think she was pretty chuffed I'd asked her to cut my hair she knew I'd only had Chris cut my hair for the last twenty plus years, but now Chris was so busy. My niece came to get the scissors and cut my hair and it's been fabulous so I will be asking her to cut it for me now just because it's easier and she did a lovely cut, I must admit I was very nervous as I'm very fussy being a hairdresser myself, my poor niece must have been scared doing it to, but she shouldn't have been and neither should I.

I'd never been to Scotland until my youngest niece Julie, married her husband David, she had a wonderful wedding in a castle, up in Sterling it was truly magical. During the night I heard a tapping at the door next door, it kept happening so I got up to tell them to be quiet but no one was there, until a little voice said, "Hello, Nanny." My three-year-old granddaughter was standing there.

I looked down and couldn't believe my eyes, I was sharing a room with my mum, she didn't hear a thing, so I put my slippers and dressing gown on and took her back to her mummy, I couldn't find the light switch so I called out to Gemma to put the light on, poor girl was fast asleep and didn't have a clue what was going on, until I told her of course, to this day we don't know if Freya managed to unlock the door.

Several years after getting married my niece Julie and David had their first child a beautiful little girl called Jessica, I find it difficult with her living in Scotland but we Facetime and keep in touch. She came down to Milton Keynes while I was in Bedford Hospital and she came to see me. Oh, it was so good to meet Jessica for the first time, she's such a clever girl – very advanced, so when I got out of hospital and I was used to sitting for longer periods I asked Gemma and my two grandchildren to take me up to see them. We stayed in a Premier Inn; it was fabulous with an adjoining room for the children too. We had a lovely visit with them, then on the Sunday we went into Edinburgh to the restaurant where my nephew is a chef. My great nephew came as well, it was lovely with all of us together as we don't get to see each other very much. We've decided to go again in October for a little longer, I think four nights next time, so we don't have to rush. It's lovely getting away with Gemma as she's my carer any way and it gives Steve a well-earned break as now, he has to do everything and look after me. I can't be left alone because I can't even go to the toilet by myself or get a drink, hopefully in time things will improve. I'm making progress with how I move and do things more independently it's just knowing how to do it. When I try and I feel safe I'm okay so one day I'm determined to be as independent as I can be and take some of the pressure off Steve, even if it's just doing the cooking!

We aren't really fans of eating out, personally I prefer what we prepare at home, I know it's good fresh, mostly healthy food. We don't really eat junk food or high-fat meals but I was really thin when I came out of hospital, everyone tells me how well I look but I think it's because I've put on lots of weight just sitting on my bum! Hopefully the stubbies will help me lose some of this weight, I can't help snacking and I know I need to stop but I get bored because I can't get up and do anything and Steve has turned into a feeder just like I used to be. I'm just not strong enough to say no, but I really should or my wheelchair won't fit soon!

As I've said before people tell me they couldn't cope with what I have been through but you have no choice. I just got on with it, it's hard sometimes I won't lie, but I'm pretty much always smiling. I have had a bad day where I have had a meltdown, if my hair's not right or I get an infection because I've had sepsis and I'm more susceptible to getting it again so I tend to go into panic mode and get really stressed, at this moment I know it's silly but I can't help it, I know it's not rational but it happens in the blink of an eye and I just loose it. I guess it's partly because I don't have hands and legs to feel cold now so I worry I wouldn't feel the symptoms but I hope, if I get it again, I'd know I'd got a temperature and I'd be shivering and the severe breathlessness and then of course the last one I noticed was my slurred speech, some people just get one symptom others might get all. Some people have different symptoms, I'm pretty sure I'd know if I had an infection and if I felt unwell, I'd definitely go straight to A&E the last time I did they were amazing I was given intravenous antibiotics after about ten minutes of arriving they were brilliant!

A while back I went to walk my dog round Furzton Lake, it's a lovely walk from my daughter's house through an underpass into Furzton, then it's almost as if you're in the countryside. You walk along a little path by the side of a stream with bushes all around, but when we crossed into Furzton I was so busy looking at someone's garden I didn't see the yellow bollard and I crashed into it. I was telling Steve to make the wheelchair go back but he did it quite quickly and bang I was on the floor; I laugh about it now but I wasn't laughing at the time. My poor bottom hit the floor with a thud, Steve luckily managed to pick me up by himself but then a man came rushing out of a house in his dressing gown and asked if he could help, Steve's first comment to me while I was on the floor was, "What are you doing down there?"

I think I said, "I wanted to sit on the floor." We carried on and walked the dog, we went all round the lake and home again. When I told Gemma, I think she was worried but thankfully I didn't hurt myself just bruised my pride a little I was lucky because it could have been worse, we often laugh about it, it's funny Gemma and I often have a bit of banter. We joke, saying "I'm always legless now."

People say, "Oh Gemma, you can't say that."

Then I say, "But it's true, look!" and point to my missing legs. I like to joke rather than mope about it, life's too short to give up, I want to live life to the full now, do things like my skydive that I wouldn't have done before I lost my limbs, defying death definitely changes your views on life and how you want to live what you have left. I could die tomorrow but at least no one will ever say I shut myself away and didn't ever help myself or do anything with my life after I lost my limbs

Chapter 9

Today I got my Gemma to take me to B&Q I didn't want Steve to take me because it gets hot at home and we don't like leaving our dog for long., I wanted some bedding plants for some pots I have. When I got them home Steve gave them a good watering as they were very dry, he left them for a while then planted them for me, once I told him what I wanted where. It's pleasant to sit outside and have some pretty flowers to look at. Tomorrow I've got a prosthetic and physio. appointment at Stanmore and my Gemma is going away for a week tomorrow I'm going to miss her looking after me, but I've got another carer who covers holiday and does two weekends a month so she's covering. Normally Gemma would take Marley, my dog home with her but she won't be here so we've decided we will take him with us and I can go in on my own while Steve takes him for a walk and then they can sit in my Motability vehicle while they wait for me. It will be cooler in there, with the air conditioning on – it's so hot in the gym at Stanmore it's beyond a joke. They really need air conditioning because they don't have windows which they can open, so with just a fan it's a nightmare for me, something I didn't know about before losing limbs but being a quadruple amputee I'm hot nearly all of the time, I rarely need heating on, I mostly sit with the door open even in the winter and Steve has his coat on!

I will literally be melting in the gym tomorrow so I normally love it but because it's so warm outside I know it will be roasting in there and I'm dreading tomorrow. I do like sitting outside under the umbrella, I have to be careful I have a lot of bad scars from the sepsis and so I can't afford to get them burnt as the skin is very thin, but even though I'm mostly in the shade occasionally I'm walking Marley with Steve so I'm getting a pleasant colour. He made me laugh yesterday when he said my legs are white and I should get them out, I asked what's the point I'm not going to lift up my skirt to show them off, it was different when I actually had normal length legs.:)

Losing your limbs makes you hot firstly because we sweat from our hands and feet and secondly because we don't have the same area for our blood to circulate but still have the same amount of blood in our bodies, I had no idea before I lost my limbs. While in Bedford Hospital I was in a private room and had the window open all the time and I had a fan on me too, only about twice I asked for the fan to be switched off but don't think I had the window shut, I guess until you're in this situation you wouldn't know, my family and I have only learned this since I lost my limbs!

It's funny how I often think about how I learned who my real friends where through contracting sepsis, and even learned about my family. I got messages and visits from hairdressing clients and yet some family didn't text or visit so I don't speak to some people now I just can't be bothered with people that aren't genuine, life's too short. I bumped into an old client today she said how well I was looking; I was lucky as lots of my clients I'd worked for twenty plus years and now they feel like friends after working for them for all that time.

I don't know if you've heard of phantom pain but I don't get it too badly in my legs anymore but my hands are horrendous most of the time it's as if I have tight clenched fists and really bad pins and needles and electric shocks mixed together. Occasionally I get a shooting pain like an electric shock and my leg jumps in the air, it's quite funny really and when I tell my grandson he says, "But you don't have legs Nanny."

Then, I tell him that my brain still thinks they are there because I had legs for a long time, he's only five so he will probably never remember me with hands and legs!

One day I was sat at the table and I was chatting with Gemma when I looked down saying the dog just tickled my foot, then we both burst out laughing I said, "But I don't have legs." We both laughed for ages it's strange at times my legs feel as if they are still there. I miss my hands so much, I can do lots of things with my stumps, like feed myself with toast or a meal with a strap on my arm or put my make-up on, I drink tea in a thermos cup so I can hold it with my stumps, the only thing I really have to be fed with is a sandwich, because I like fillings like tomato with ham and the sandwich ends up falling apart, but I want to do it myself so I will find a way. Today I sat up by myself for the first time, when my daughter arrived she didn't believe that I had done it and I thought that I couldn't do it again but after my shower I lay on the bed while she was dressing me and managed to sit up I think she was surprised too, it certainly feels good to be doing more for myself.

I never knew how hard it could be to go on holiday, or anywhere new, when you are a quadruple amputee. I can't just book a normal room it has to be adapted you don't think of these things so I find a hotel then I have to ring them to check it's fully accessible with a wet room, I just didn't think about these things before. Recently I went to Manchester to go on the Jeremy Kyle Show and although the hotel was fine, the bed was so uncomfortable I kept trying to move and was groaning so much, Gemma asked what was wrong and I told her that it was the bed. I wanted to get in my wheelchair, it wasn't great sleeping in my wheelchair but it was better than that bed. The next morning, I told the male receptionist. I guessed he was from Spain so I spoke to him, in Spanish, of course, we had a little Spanish chat, it was so good to practice my Spanish, I used to talk it to a group of the Spanish nurses in Bedford Hospital. I love the language, I get by quite well, I'm hoping one day I will be able to go back and visit our friends but at the moment I'm too scared. My girls don't want me to go back either but I do miss the culture and the friends we have there, I miss trying to speak the language, I used to meet with Spanish ladies who wanted to speak English so we would talk for half an hour in English and half an hour Spanish it was great because we would help each other, having a coffee sitting in the sun, I miss that. It was good having time to relax in Spain, I hope I feel okay to go back one day, I'm getting stronger and more confident, but if I flew I'd either have to have a wheelchair-accessible vehicle over there so I could take my electric wheelchair or I'd have to take my manual and be pushed around. I would hate that as I lose my independence then, and I like to be as independent as I can be!

Chapter 10

So today I went to Stanmore again and stood for a bit longer, it's so strange I was really wobbly, the physio. explained to me why I was so wobbly – our bodies automatically tip us backwards and so you end up leaning forward to counter that. Also we never stand 100% still our feet keep us balanced, not having feet my hips are doing that, I think she's said there are twenty-six joints in the feet with muscles all around them but I just have my hips and the big muscles behind them so it takes a lot of getting used to.

I can tell you, I was probably only standing for a minute but it was so tiring so I had to lean on the plinth, but I was able to keep doing it and even managed to let go, it was just so good I'm buzzing to think that hopefully by Christmas I'll actually be walking again.

Another achievement, which I've managed three times in the last few days, is to sit up by myself, it might sound silly but I literally have to learn how to do everything again, it's not easy and it's not something that happens overnight but I'm happy with my progress so far, it is hard work but I'm not scared about that. I'm prepared to put in the work to get my independence back and slowly I am, I'm prepared for the long haul.

We took Marley with us to Stanmore today, as I'm confident enough to go in on my own, but in case the door was closed, which it often is, Steve came to open it.

He went outside to Marley, I had to laugh when the receptionist asked, "Is he in the dog house today?"

I replied saying, "No he's in the bus with the dog." He was actually sitting on the bench and took Marley for a nice walk, he was so good, bless him, I was just glad it was sunny and not raining as we had him with us.

I found out today that they don't normally give you rehabilitation with a private limb, so they've discussed it and as long as I'm happy for them to not touch my Open Bionics Hero Arm, and I take any responsibility if it breaks, they will give me rehab. I took out a five-year accidental insurance on it so I said, "It's not a problem." I'm happy they would still help me.

Unfortunately, I can't make physio. next week because my daughter Becki is taking me to the school where she teaches to go in their hydrotherapy pool, I'm really excited about this, but I'm going to Stanmore afterwards to meet with the OT to practice in the kitchen with my Hero Arm. I can't wait to see what gadgets and tips she can give me to help me start cooking again, I'm not sure what I'm most excited about cooking or walking! Both, equally, I think.

Just been thinking, because my back's hurting tonight, I hope my slipped discs and the arthritis in my back and hips don't stop me from walking, as long as I can walk indoors at least once a day I'll be happy, I'm not to bothered if I can't stay walking all day every day. That wasn't my reason for legs in the first place but hopefully I will be able to do more than just a little bit. At rehab. I've seen people achieve so much, including myself, they really are amazing at helping you do what you need to do. Some of the my exercises I have to do are when either sitting or lying I have to draw my hip up towards my armpit, that is how I will have to walk by lifting the hip to lift and move my leg, a big learning curve as I also have to keep my balance it's really not easy, it takes an awful lot of energy and concentration.

I just hope I can have enough energy for it as just standing for a minute takes a lot of energy and I'm not ready to start walking yet, I was told this will take me, as an bilateral-above-knee amputee, between 75% and 80% more energy than it did when I had legs! That's a massive amount more energy, I think I'll be going for a sleep once I've walked a short distance at first!

I went to the dentist a few days ago and on the wall was a poster about Safeguarding, it brought back an unwelcome memory. This was when I had a carer, who I had thought was really pleasant, made me feel extremely uncomfortable when she was washing me down below it just didn't feel right. I cried all day it really upset me so I phoned the care company and told them not to send her to me ever again. I just didn't want to see her again or to ever feel like that again. This also reminded me of when I was in Roehampton Hospital and a nurse came in to our ward, there were only four beds and I asked her to close the curtain as I needed to have a wee. I was using a female urinal as I couldn't get on the toilet and the nurse said, "No one is around so it is okay." And she wouldn't shut the curtain.

I said, "Kelly is up, she's in the bathroom." But the nurse still insisted that no one was up as she hadn't seen anyone. But she sat at a table along the corridor from our ward so, of course she didn't see anyone. Next I was in the middle of having a wee, when Kelly stuck her head in to say hello. I was mortified I screamed at the nurse, "Now do you believe me, now will you close the curtain?"

I lost it big time, I asked her, "Do you go in a public toilet and leave the door open? Am I not allowed dignity?" I cried all day, I didn't go to the gym, I wouldn't eat, I was devastated and I didn't even get an apology!

I've been through so much I'm surprised I'm still sane but I pick myself up and dust myself off and get on with life. I get comments all the time about how inspirational I am and how I'm always smiling but that's just my way, I think giving the talks about sepsis is why I'm still alive, I'm strong always have been, and giving the talks helps me to heal in so many ways. I emailed a man I met in hospital a few days ago and heard back from him today he had meningococcal septicaemia and was the first ever quadruple amputee I'd ever met. I didn't know any before I lost my limbs, Mike his name is, today I heard back from him, we've been keeping in touch since leaving hospital via email it's good to see what he's been up to, he was amazing. When he heard that I was in hospital he came and found me and chatted, it was good to be able to talk to someone who knew what I was going through. He was a little ahead of me with his rehab., he gives talks warning people about meningitis and sepsis, he also said he finds it has helped him heal. I have emailed him to tell him about my Hero Arm and that Open Bionics had been to film me with it, he was happy to hear about everything.

Chapter ll

Since becoming a quadruple amputee, myself I've met a few others, children and adults, they have all had meningococcal septicaemia unlike me. My sepsis was from a kidney infection. Mike only had one kidney and was on dialysis for some months but luckily his kidney is working enough and he doesn't have to have dialysis anymore. I was so lucky as it was only a week after getting sepsis that my kidneys kicked back in, it's funny I often think about how lucky I am. Lots of people wouldn't think they were lucky if they were in my situation, but I am because I'm alive and have my amazing family who help me. My husband is becoming an excellent cook and carer, he looks after me so well. It is not something I ever expected he'd have to do but he just got on with it even though it must have been so hard for him. My eldest daughter used to be a carer and my youngest teaches special needs children so they've both worked in caring jobs and they are both brilliant with me. My sister Sheryl, visits once a week and does my ironing, I'm putting money away for her. And my mum will do anything if I ask her, she's so good I'm so very lucky!

I won't lie, life is more challenging now. If I have times when I think that I can't do something then I'll maybe think about it and try to do it in a way which I think might work and often it does. I just have to learn to do things all over again often in a very different way. My family try to protect me from things and at times I have to tell them to let me do some things, it's my way of learning rather in the same way that babies do, it's hard but I'm not a quitter.

If this book gets read by a hundred people and they all tell one friend and that friend tells a friend and it saves just one person's life I'd be so happy. All of those who have had sepsis affect us badly want others to be aware of sepsis and meningitis, slowly everyone is hearing about these illnesses and hopefully they will remember the symptoms and that will save lives. This means so much to me. If I can help to save lives then me being a quadruple amputee and what happened to me will be worth it. All that I'm going to go through and the struggle I'll probably have for the rest of my life, will be worth it. So, I'm very lucky to have a family who help me to give the talks and spread awareness of sepsis

At the special needs school where my daughter Becki teaches, they have a hydrotherapy swimming pool, Becki took me there during the half term break, I was able to stand up and practice walking. I also managed to do lots of exercises that I'd done a few weeks before with the OTs at Stanmore it was so good. Becki said that she thought I'd be allowed to go in once a week after school and during the summer half term, but unfortunately there was a huge disappointment – due to a problem with the roof no one is allowed in there now, I'm gutted for the children it must be so hard for all of them!

I keep getting phantom pain in my legs, it's not painful as such, but it's so strange I had osteoarthritis and was getting close to needing a knee replacement in my left knee before I lost my legs and I keep getting pain as if my knee is still there and hurting. I've been getting a lot of electric shocks again in my feet, my grandson doesn't understand when I say my foot's hurting. He always says, "But you don't have feet."

I always tell him, "But I had feet for a very long time and my brain still thinks they are there and tries to make me think they are there by giving me signals of pain, playing tricks with me." Mostly I try to cope with it by ignoring it as much as possible I find it helps!

I'm still working hard to contact people and companies to give talks about sepsis, I had a call last night from a lady who has been messaging me following a post I'd put on Facebook about giving talks. We chatted for a while, she's now going to work to find some possible dates and email them to me so that I can choose which will be best for me. I will never give up trying to spread awareness about sepsis, I really feel it's why I didn't die and that I can help saves lives. I'm really passionate about people knowing about sepsis and how it's turned my, and my family's lives life upside down. It's been horrendous but although life is a challenge now it is one I can cope with, it definitely helps me to talk about what happened and to warn people.

I'm struggling recently with back pain, since going to Stanmore not long ago and standing on my stubbies, I have osteoarthritis in all my joints and my back and I have three slipped discs in my back. I know the pain is because I stood for a time and I'm really not sure it's going to be possible now, I'm hoping it will settle but

I don't want to have to take painkillers just to be able to walk and then to suffer for weeks afterwards hopefully it will settle and it's just a hiccough.

I was really hoping to be walking by Christmas I haven't spoken to the staff at Stanmore about it yet because I'm still hoping it will be okay so I'm keeping my options open.

Earlier, I was thinking about my family, as I often do, and how hard it must have been for them, especially in the first few weeks. But to go on for nine weeks not knowing and having the language barrier in Spain to cope with as well. Thank goodness for our Spanish friend who used to translate for Steve, he gave some updates a little. But I do wonder what sort of care I got in Spain especially as I arrived back with the pressure sores, my head looked like it had split in half and you could see my skull it was so bad, it was still being dressed while I was in Roehampton more than five months after coming back from Spain!

Doctors and nurses couldn't believe how bad it was, it was so sore to lie on it too, I'm very lucky. I've got a T section that hasn't got hair now and it never will have, but I've grown the layers a little longer just enough to cover it, so unless I want to show someone you can't actually see it now. My family were very upset seeing it in Milton Keynes Hospital as I had to show my daughters everything when they met me. Then for a further three weeks they were with me every day waiting for me to wake up, once the medication which was keeping me in a coma was stopped they didn't think it looked good, because I didn't wake when they expected me to, I think I was enjoying the sleep to be honest.:)

But gradually I did come round, I remember one day, when they put something over the tracheostomy in my throat so I could talk, the girls took a video of me – it's quite funny to watch. They kept saying "You can talk now Mum." I just stared at them as if they were speaking a foreign language I didn't speak, I think I might have nodded but don't remember talking. I remember when they took my tracheotomy out, I wasn't allowed to drink but my mouth was really dry so I was allowed little sips of water but had to spit them out. I would take a bigger sip and swallow a little, my girls knew what I'd done and would tell me off. I knew I was okay and I love cold water I couldn't resist it. Once I had woken up on Ward 2 there was a drinking fountain that gave really cold water, it was fabulous once I was allowed to drink, I drank gallons of it, then it broke – I was devastated!

I didn't like Ward 2 as I was supposed to have three nurses taking care of me if I needed moving for anything but one nurse took it upon herself to move me on her own, she didn't care if she hurt me or anything, she was horrible. I'll never forget her; I often wonder if she still works there. I'd like to go to Ward 2 one day and see, because I've got a few things I'd like to say to her! I think about the night I had to get the male HCA to phone my daughters because of an uncaring nurse. I hope the matron dealt with that nurse. I hope she was sacked for everything she did, she didn't like that I complained about her dealing with me 1:1 instead of 3:1 as she should have done. After that she did other things like mess with medication and other things. She got staff listening to her, I think she must have told them that if they didn't do as she said they wouldn't work in Milton Keynes Hospital again and they must have believed her. She got two nurses who were changing bandages on my legs to leave me, they said they had to go for their break but would be back but I saw them with their coats leaving. My girls came in and I told them they had to get someone else to come and redress my legs and change my sheets because the dressings hadn't been changed properly and my legs bleeding and weeping on the sheets, it was pretty horrendous. I wouldn't wish anyone to lose their job but when she's in a caring profession and she treats a patient the way she treated me she deserved to lose her job.

The matron was lovely she kept coming and checking on me and had someone she trusted sit in my room with me that night. This was after I got the male HCA to phone my girls for me, I don't think he believed me about this Kirsten at first but after I told him a few things he called my girls I was so grateful. The uncaring nurse knew I'd refused male carers, I didn't want a man anywhere near me to change me or anything I just wanted ladies, she made a point of bringing him in and saying, "If Kim needs changing, you're okay with that aren't you?"

I couldn't believe my ears I was devastated; I would have laid in a wet bed all night rather than let a man see my bits, I've always been a private person and shy about my body I would have died if he'd have done anything.

Thankfully I didn't have to worry once my girls arrived along with the matron, they got me calmed down and sorted, but again I had a bit of a hallucinatory moment about this, because I thought I was taken upstairs to the flat of matron's friend. I thought that she was packing for her holiday and my friend's son came to take her to the airport, that was certainly an hallucination because I was still in the side room on Ward 2!

Strange really how being in a coma for so long with all the drugs I'd been pumped with I really believed these things – particularly this hallucination and that my husband was gay. The bit I'd have liked to have been true was that we were going to Australia to have a barbeque on the beach, now how nice would that have been with all my family?

I've recently booked a couple of holidays with my daughter and the grandchildren, one in August this year to go to Holland to visit a family that are like our family now. Their daughter Nathalie, came to live with us seven years ago to study at a local school, she was so clever top of the year in every subject and was so lovely we never had any problems with her. Her family came over for a holiday even though they weren't supposed to while the children were with us but Nathalie assured us that she wouldn't be wanting to go home, which she didn't. I invited the family for a meal at our house and then, for a celebration to surprise Nathalie when it was her eighteenth. They'd booked a flight but her dad wanted a coffee and missed boarding so they ended up driving over from the Netherlands, her mum Lillian, wasn't happy and I knew I'd have been the same.

They made it okay and we had a lovely time, Nathalie was so surprised as we hadn't told her a thing, her parents are coming to see us next week, we are meeting and going out for a meal. We haven't seen them since just before I lost my limbs but they know all about it, we keep in touch and Gemma and the children are looking forward to taking me to Holland to see them.

The last time I went Steve and I took Freya; she loved it and is looking forward to going again. We went while Nathalie was living with us so that's about six years ago so it's going to be lovely going back again. I chose a hotel that looked okay but I needed to be sure so I spoke to Nathalie and she phoned the hotel to check I would be given a disabled room with a room next door, that way Freya can sleep in my room and if I need anything (which I don't normally during the night) she can go and get Gemma.

Our next break is in October when we are going up to Scotland to visit family again, I think Steve likes Gemma taking me away because he gets a break. I know looking after me is hard work, occasionally he upsets me, he doesn't mean to but when I need help to go to the toilet, I can't go by myself and need help. When he tuts and sighs and asks, "Are you trying to kill me?" I can't help but get upset. I've always been a very independent woman and have never asked anyone to do things for me but I have no choice now because I rely on everyone to help me and I have to ask, I hope one day I can do more for myself.

I'm looking forward to seeing my family in Scotland again especially my great niece and great nephew. Tom is sixteen now and it seems like only yesterday he was a baby; the years have flown. I miss him as he lives in Scotland. Jessica she's two she's my niece's daughter Tom is my nephew's son they are lovely children but living so far away we don't get to see each other as much as I'd like. Julie and David come down sometimes. My nephew James is a chef so sadly he doesn't come down very much so I hope I'll get to see him again when I'm up there.

Chapter 12

Gemma is taking me to New York in February 2020 I can't wait it's always somewhere I've wanted to go but Steve doesn't like the idea of a long-haul flight so he told Gemma to take me and he'd look after the grandchildren, bless him. Now I'm really looking forward to seeing so many places we are staying in Times Square so we will be close to everything and I want to visit the Empire State Building, The Statue of Liberty, Central Park a Broadway show. I told my mum I'd like to see a show she said that by the end of a day of sightseeing she would be falling asleep so maybe I'll have to see if I think I'll be okay, I guess as I won't be walking anywhere I won't be tired.:)

I can't wait to see the shops and high-rise buildings and of course Ground Zero that will be amazing as I'm sure I'll be blown away by how massive the site is. It's always seemed quite small to me on TV but it's got to be huge with it being such a big building, we've bought passes to get to see as much as possible and being in Times Square I know everything is fairly close. I'm sure the Americans are good with disabled facilities better than the UK I'm sure, but I worry everywhere I go. With hotels I always check that I'll have a wet room and that it's wheelchair accessible but also for toilets because of my wheelchair the toilet has to be big enough for me to get in.

For his birthday in February we took Steve to the Chelsea football grounds for a tour and afterwards we went to the London Eye. We decided to go to a cafe for some lunch, I need the loo so we asked, but my goodness it was a joke, there were staff lockers in there, buckets, mops all kinds of stuff, it was so full I had a job to get in. You don't think about these things until you need them but a disabled toilet shouldn't be used as a store cupboard it made it very difficult for me to get in.

Hopefully America is set up for disability better they are bigger and better at most things, I've been to America many times over the years my real dad lived there most of his life, in Texas. My last visit was after he passed away five years ago this December just before Christmas. My girls and I went one last time to clear his house so it could be sold I had to see his lawyer with his will and deal with things, they certainly are such lovely people. The first time I went to visit him in Texas was when he went back there to live. He returned to the UK for ten years and during his first or second year he was involved in a road rage incident, he jumped out of his car and the other guy drove straight at him. Luckily, he jumped between the driver's door onto the bonnet but sadly his leg was smashed. He waited a very long time but after about eight years got compensation, with that money he brought a trailer park and a bar in Midland Texas, I liked it there but when he died, he was living in small town called Blackwell. The nearest town, Sweetwater was where we stayed this was thirty-two miles away and that's where his lawyer was too. We had to go thirty-four miles the other way from where my dad had lived to the funeral parlour to collect the paperwork, they have wonderful, big roads out there and you don't see much traffic unless you're in a big city.

The first time I took my girls to America my dad drove us from Texas to Florida. As a single parent of young children, I didn't know if I'd ever be able to afford to visit again. My dad gave us all £2,000 each, my sister, myself and all five grandchildren. That was an awful lot of money back in 1991 so I decided to go and visit Dad's new home and Florida. We went to Disneyland; it was amazing and I'll never forget it. It was long drive I think it took about thirty-two hours and we only stopped for fuel, food or to use the toilet. It was such a long drive that I don't know how he did it. I couldn't have driven that far without a break as it took nine hours just to get out of Texas. We used the biggest motorway I've ever seen which was in Houston, it had ten lanes and it was packed. On the way back we hit it at the busiest time but what an experience. I remember he wouldn't let me help with the driving and I was glad as I'd have been a bit scared. Most of the way we saw hardly any traffic, but he always got me to look out for a roof rack as cop cars had roof racks on and would sit waiting for speeding cars, he rarely went over the speed limit but you still had to be careful.

Texans are lovely and my dad was a character, I didn't really know him until he came back from America when I was twenty-one. He and my mum split when I was eight, my mum met someone else and they married when I was eleven. This man was wonderful, he took us on as his own, he had never had children of his own and we always called him dad. He was our dad he did everything for us, my real dad didn't even give my mum any money, rarely phoned to talk to us or to ask my mum how we were, he just got on with his life like a young single man without any worries. He had fun and women friends. It's sad that someone who led the life he did died a very lonely old man with nothing, and my step dad led a good life and died at just fifty-four, suddenly in the night with a heart attack. It's sad he isn't here to see the grandchildren and great grandchildren he'd have loved them all. He was amazing we all miss him so much even now; it broke my heart when he died – so very sad. I'm going to be fifty-eight in July and I don't feel old. I think you realise how short life is especially surviving death, like I have and being older than the age my dad was when he died.

I've booked a cruise for February 2021 I know it's a long way off but it's the year of my sixtieth and we wanted to go away for it. I found this cruise; we've always wanted to go to Portugal and see more of Spain the cruise goes to several places in Spain and to Portugal on the way home. It's going to be wonderful; I've always wanted to go to Barcelona and that is just one of the stops I'm looking forward to. We went on our first cruise last November; Steve has never wanted to take a cruise but I've always wanted to. Now I can't do our normal beach holidays anymore this will be great for me. We went on a four-day cruise to Belgium which was nice we got off the boat and had a look around the shops, we had a coffee and the next day were supposed to land in Amsterdam but sadly it was too windy so we couldn't dock.

We had a sea day, but it was okay we walked around the ship, looked around the shops, watched a film, sat and had a coffee and chatted with other people. We went with P&O and I would recommend them any time, they certainly look after you especially disabled people. That is why we booked with them again, the food was amazing everything you wanted and more the service was the best I've ever had. Although Steve had to care for me, he still enjoyed his time away, that's why we've booked to go again I think it's the best holiday I've ever had, and I've had some lovely holidays in my life. I've always worked very hard for my holidays, because I worked so hard, I needed beach holidays to relax and unwind reading a book, I enjoy reading, I hate it when I am enjoying a good read and I get to the end of the book. I think it's a good book when you want more!

I was reading a book on my Kindle before I went in the coma, I didn't pick my Kindle up again until a few months ago, and when I started reading it again the story came back to me after a couple of pages. It was about the First World War it was such a good book, it made me think of my grandad he fought in the Second World War, and he didn't see my mum until she was three years old, it makes you think about how tough it was for them back then, it brings me back to thinking of how my family coped.

Steve would have been lost, I did everything all paying of bills, cooking and housework, if he put the Hoover round he always said, "I've done your housework for you." Ha, ha as if it's that easy, bless him, he did the cars and the garden, we worked well doing our own jobs, but when I was in a coma, he didn't know how to get money from the bank or anything, thank goodness my Becki's really good and helped him. And thanks to her for finding my travel insurance and getting me home, where

I belong with my amazing family around me, I think the worry has aged them all, especially my poor mum, I feel so bad about what I have put them all through nine whole weeks of not knowing if I'd live or die.

Even when I was taken off the drugs that were keeping me in the coma it took a long time for me to wake up even then they didn't think I was going to put through, at one point my face had dropped and they thought I'd had a stroke so I had to have a scan to check, thankfully it was okay. I had pneumonia and had to have a couple of X-rays because of that I certainly tested them, and although Spain just about kept me alive I believe Milton Keynes DOCC saved my life, I'm so very grateful for that. The treatment and the amputations that have saved my life and for my rehabilitation at Roehampton and now at Stanmore without all that I think I'd be dead now I've literally had to learn how to do everything again. Sitting up was so hard, I remember thinking I'll never be able to do this, but gradually I learned how to balance to sit then the physiotherapists used to try pushing me from side to side to see if I was steady and it took a long time, mainly because I only saw them once a week. I certainly didn't get as much physio. in Bedford as I'd have liked after my amputations, so when I got to Roehampton and I had to go to the gym all day with a break for lunch, I expected to be really tired but I was fine. I learned how to shuffle on my bottom up and down the plinth, I remember thinking I can't do this and then thinking, go on you can do it and all of a sudden, I was doing it. The physios were very pleased with my progress and all the time telling me how I was doing more than they expected so quickly, but like I've said before I've always been hard working and don't quit, it was just getting myself to realise what I had to do to move, like with learning to walk again and being able to get my balance and then learning to lift at the hip to then move my legs, it's going to be hard and I really hope my back will be able to let me walk again!

Chapter 13

On Mother's Day, 2018 I was in Bedford Hospital and my girls were simply amazing I cried lots of happy tears because my grandson was allowed in. This was unusual but they made an exception and we had a picnic on my bed, we had sandwiches, sausage rolls, pork pies, cakes and more it was so lovely. Becki is so thoughtful planning things like that and because I'm not allowed fresh flowers in hospital, they brought me a beautiful green metal bucket which said 'Flowers' on it filled with beautiful silk flowers. The nurses thought they were real and asked them to take them home, they didn't believe they artificial. Due to the coma, the medication and the sepsis my memory was really poor, I still struggle at times but it's a lot better than it was, they really spoilt me with lots of gifts and I think it's the best Mother's Day I've ever had it was more special than anything.

My girls have been my life, I've always helped them and been there to support them, we are a close family and I thank God we are. I really don't think I would have got through this without them, my Gemma is my main carer and if I don't see her (as I haven't recently because she has just had her first holiday as a single parent) I miss her. I had another carer and it was the first time Gemma has had a week off since she started being my carer. I'm used to the way Gemma does things, so when someone else takes over it's all new to them too, they've probably never dealt with an amputee never mind a quadruple amputee. I'm really fussy and like things done a certain way, and thankfully the replacement, Alison, was great – I'm nervous of carers after the care company I had when I first came out of hospital!

Alison is lovely and so gentle so we will get on fine, but I missed Gemma so much while she was on holiday. My Becki came and took me out with my daughter-in-law Sam, we went to Dobbies where I helped choose plants for them for their garden. They've recently had some work done and a new fence, she's now planted her plants and the garden is looking lovely, I don't see as much of Becki now as she works long hours and is also a cake-maker. She makes the most amazing cakes and has a massive talent; I totally understand she can't come that often but she makes time for me nevertheless and I really appreciate our time together.

It's all the more special when we have time together, like going for lunch or even just going to the garden centre it's lovely getting out doing something different and spending time with my girls and my grandchildren is wonderful. I love it when the grandchildren come to stay, they love being with us too, Oliver is getting better with Steve who just loves to wind him up and Oliver listens to me when Steve starts now, instead of taking notice of grandad.

I've always had such a special bond with my grandchildren I was there at Freya's birth it was the most amazing experience ever, she's such a lovely kind girl, nothing is too much trouble for her if I ask her to do something for me, she's a sweetheart. Making memories with them, going to Holland and Scotland is wonderful I feel very privileged to be able to spend so much time with them, we have had some wonderful times over the years. Oliver doesn't remember when I had hands and legs now, so he will just have to look at pictures when he's older to see how I used to look. This normal to him now, Freya remembers but I'm not sure she will in years to come as she's only ten now!

I remember Becki telling me that they were waiting for me to arrive back from Spain waiting outside the DOCC they got excited but, I can only imagine, scared as well, when they saw a trolley being wheeled down the corridor, they couldn't see if it was me but they knew it must be. I was wrapped in what looked like a body bag and they were relieved that I was finally back with them in the UK.

In my post rehab. review, the consultant told me just how ill I'd been when they received me back and how serious things were, how bleak it looked then. He actually told me he was surprised to see me looking so well! He was lovely telling me all about my care and asking questions about how I was feeling. He asked if I had flashbacks but thankfully I didn't, I was suffering from an extremely bad memory and we did joke about my hallucinations he told me lots about things I didn't know. He told me that the infection in my body had caused my immune system to go into overdrive turning to sepsis, which then caused septicaemia and then septic shock, it was the first time I'd been told this and I was fascinated. He explained that was why I'd had to have the kidney dialysis as septic shock is when vital organs start shutting down, to try to save the organs the body stops sending blood to the extremities like hands and feet. This is why my hands and legs went black and I had to have the amputations, I appreciated him explaining everything to me. All I knew was that they'd gone black and needed to be removed but didn't know the reason other than sepsis had caused it. I didn't understand what sepsis was then. Lots of people think you can catch sepsis but that's not true. It can be any infection at all, from a simple paper cut to a UTI, any infection can cause our immune system to go into overdrive it's an extreme reaction to any infection and so anyone can get sepsis. Much more work and training needs to be carried out to increase awareness, I'm passionate about trying to warn people about sepsis now.

I'm always being told I'm inspirational, I'm just me, strong independent and stubborn well I was independent I'm not so independent now, but I try to be. For example, this week I have achieved being able to go across from my wheelchair to my bed more independently. I thought I'd like to try doing it without the banana board I normally use because of the six-inch gap, so I told Steve I'd got an idea and wanted to try it. It was a success so I can now do it without the banana board which makes me a little more independent which certainly feels good!

My Becki has found it all very hard, she doesn't talk about these things with me but I know when it's an anniversary of something like my amputations she'll tell me this happened a year ago today by text and a crying face. She doesn't like to see pictures of my black limbs; I know these upset her even though she doesn't always say. I feel it's good to share them to help people to be aware of what sepsis can do. This has more impact than just hearing the word sepsis. People can get to know what causes it, the symptoms so that everyone understands and is aware. I post often trying to warn people, I can't rest I don't want others suffering like my family and I have, or worse dying. It kills so quickly, sometimes we don't like to bother the GP or the hospital just because we feel a little unwell. For myself I think I knew I was very unwell but the language barrier didn't help, I couldn't tell them enough but then I didn't know about sepsis and that my cold hands and feet, my severe breathlessness and my slurred speech and shivering were all symptoms of sepsis – I just felt really ill.

Everyone tells me how well I look now and I feel well, I'm doing well with things I'm gradually getting more independence I'm busy trying to fundraise for another Hero Arm and I use this is Just Giving page https://www.justgiving.com/crowdfunding/kim-smith-3. I've got a long way to go but I've got one and I'm happy with the independence that gives me for now. The Hero Arm from Open Bionics truly is amazing, it has so much more functionality than my NHS prosthetic arm and it is so much lighter which makes it so much easier to use. I can't hold the NHS one up for long without my arm getting very tired.

When I was in hospital and when I first came home, I didn't sleep much. I often didn't go to sleep until 2 or 3 a.m. or I'd go to sleep around midnight and wake at about 4 a.m., luckily I managed to buy an iPad Pro with my fundraising money so once my daughter Becki bought it to me in the hospital, I'd ask the nurses to put the TV on for me (I couldn't do it with bandages on my arms). It was wonderful when the first arm had healed and I could use the iPad. Becki had set up the Kim's Chance page on Facebook and the girls would both post things to tell everyone how I was getting on, it was great when I could start doing that myself and telling everyone what I was doing sharing videos of me shuffling up my bed etc. Proud moments!

When I got home from hospital it became apparent to me that our German Shepherd dog Molly, was too much for me although she did get calmer, she would get very excited to see me and although she was still a puppy at two years old, she was big and almost tipped my wheelchair over. While we were living at Gemma's it wasn't so difficult to give the dog lots of long walks because Gemma would be at home with me while Steve walked the dogs but I realised he wouldn't be able to do that when we got into our bungalow as I can't be left for long, our Bichon Frisée is okay he only needs a little walk not like Molly. So, I looked into rehoming her with the German Shepherd Dog Rescue, they were amazing and found Molly a new home. Although it broke our hearts Steve's and I knew it was the right thing for Molly even though it would have been so easy to keep her but that would have been selfish of us. The couple who she was rehomed by had children and Molly was wonderful with children and they'd had German Shepherd dogs before. Molly had such a wonderful nature and was such a lovely girl we both miss her so much but it was kinder to let her go to a family who have got time to walk her, I'm sure she's very happy with them, I will always miss her though and I blame sepsis for taking my baby and my limbs!

Chapter 14

My sister Sheryl, has been amazing. I needed my ironing doing as not having hands I can't do it now, I asked her if she would help and she comes every week to do it for me. She's hoping to move soon so every time she's done my ironing. I have transferred money to my mum's account to save towards new carpets or whatever Sheryl needs, she wouldn't take payment for the ironing and this will come in very handy for her. I would have had to pay someone to iron for me as I would never have expected anyone to do work for free. Sheryl doesn't earn much as she's disabled herself so every little helps. She's great any time I need anything she helps and my mum is now seventy-six, seventy-seven next month and she's fitter than both me and my sister and she looks so young too we always get asked if we are sisters, my mum loves that! But if I've got her great looks when I'm her age (if I live that long) I'll be very happy she's a brilliant help too. I told her recently I wanted a rhubarb crumble so I know she'll make me one and bring it round soon, she's a diamond. I got my work ethic from her, she's always worked very hard, especially when my real dad left her and didn't give her any money. You didn't get benefits years ago like you do now, she didn't get any help and this is where I got it from. My ex. didn't give me any money, I don't know if he thought if he didn't see his daughters he didn't need to pay, I didn't want his money but it would have been good if he'd brought the girls a gift now and again or sent them some pocket money now and again. The Child Support Agency was introduced and I did think it might be fantastic and I might get some money but because he had a friend who said he worked for him for next to nothing he didn't have to pay!

Years later he started working and he was made to pay a little bit he didn't pay much or for long so it's a good job I never relied on it. I put money into my girl's savings, for them when they were older, we were lucky as Steve came into our lives, he's been an amazing step dad and husband he needs a medal for putting up with me since I've come out of hospital, he's been amazing. I'm very demanding. He's brilliant at cooking now, but I guide him telling him what to put in and how to do it, friends came for dinner a few weeks ago and were very impressed with his cooking skills!

Which is why it will be nice when we go on our cruise, two weeks of no cooking he's going to love that.:) He's quite a shy person really but he'll talk to anyone and you can't get away once he starts, he's so friendly and loves going out for meals. Whereas I'd rather stay at home, I prefer home cooked food, depending on where we go, I don't always enjoy eating out and think I'd rather save the money, not that we go out very often it's a rare treat!

I've always loved cooking and I miss it now but talking Steve through what to cook and how to is almost like I'm doing it myself which is not so bad. I used to like baking too, I was always making cakes I'd brought myself a lovely Kenwood food mixer with my tips from my hairdressing clients at Christmas. I always saved the tips and brought something nice for myself with the money. I would tell my clients what I brought too; I think it was nice to tell them what I'd put the money towards. ne year I brought a sewing machine. Steve said, "Why have you brought that? You won't use it." But I proved him wrong I used it a lot and loved it, my mum has it now and Becki has my food mixer, hopefully she can use it alongside hers when she has lots of cakes to make!

We've got Becki and Sam's dog today, he's lovely. I love having him for the day when they are working, he's so lovely and it's great for my Marley to have his playmate here they love each other and play so well together it's wonderful to watch them chasing and playing. They love being together you can see the excitement in them when they see each other they run to greet each other with their tales wagging it's nice we can help look after him.

I have a very small garden at my bungalow and I have had it all put to slabs because when we moved in the paving stones were all broken and there was a big step down, so it was not wheelchair friendly. I know of a brilliant man who has done work for us before so I phoned him and asked for a quote. I asked about bringing the paving up higher so I could get out but he said it would go above our damp-proof course and recommended putting a ramp by the door which he would do with the slabs, problem solved. He did an amazing job, I've just got a couple of pots out there and it's lovely to look out onto we've got some bits on the fence too, we love our little bungalow it's very cosy.

Finally, I want to thank my two daughters Gemma and Becki my mum, sister and husband you've always been so supportive since this happened and I'm truly grateful.

Please now you've read this be aware of any infection and if you think you have any symptoms get urgent medical attention. Do not wait, it's serious and if left you could die, if medical staff don't listen just ask, "Could it be sepsis?" be insistent that they do tests if you feel really unwell!
#sepsisawareness saves lives!

07855946919
https://m.facebook.com/Kims-Chance-1506708116112720/

CPSIA information can be obtained
at www.ICGtesting.com
Printed in the USA
BVHW080118020822
643541BV00007B/840